Dirty Talk

I0090368

The Comprehensive Handbook For Provocative And Sensual Inquiries To Enhance Intimacy, And Accessories To Elevate Your Evening

Daryl Morrow

TABLE OF CONTENT

Keep In Mind...Achieving Optimal Sexual Experiences Requires A Methodical Approach

In order to experience incredible sexual pleasure, it is necessary to explore and stimulate each erotic zone comprehensively. Though bypassing a phase may still provide enjoyment, it is imperative to note that this book is exclusively focused on transcendent, unforgettable sexual experiences. Our objective lies in exploring the type of intimacy that elicits intense sensations, causing a ripple effect through your entire being, compelling even the slightest hairs on your neck to stand on end and sending tremors of pleasure coursing through your legs.

Gaining a comfort level with discussing explicit matters requires possessing self-

1

assurance. We are referring to a level of self-assurance capable of influencing various aspects of your daily life beyond the realm of sexual experiences. Attain mastery in the domain of intimacy, and the complexities of the world appear notably less formidable.

When one possesses the assurance to assume responsibility for their own delight, they embark upon a realm characterized by elegance, fortitude, and beauty, which none can dispute, regardless of gender. Confidence is sexy. It emanates from every pore and permeates the ambitions of those in your vicinity. Embrace these explicit conversation illustrations and embark upon a journey of intense mental and physical stimulation, venturing into realms that will exceed your prior expectations.

Zone 2 for Sexual Communication – Initiating Intimate Interactions

The Preliminary Stage is the moment when the intensity arises. This is the point at which we transition from cognitive stimulation to a convergence of cognitive and physical stimulation. At this stage, he should be eagerly anticipating the opportunity to engage with you. Elevate the level of ardor by engaging in provocative conversation now that you have come together.

Utilize the provided illustrations to enhance the allure and emotional intensity as you and your partner commence engaging in intimate physical interactions. The combination of the timbre of your voice, coupled with caressing and embracing his physique, will greatly arouse his senses and intensify his response. The amalgamation will induce in him a strong urge to detonate. Continue to increase the anticipation and he will express a strong desire to engage with you intimately.

Instances of Erotic Communication Techniques Employed During Sexual Anticipation

I kindly request that you shower me with tender kisses, embracing every inch of my physique. From the sensory input received by my auditory organs, descending through my cervical region, and extending the full length of my abdominal cavity. Subsequently, I would appreciate it if you could bestow kisses upon every aspect of my thighs. Once I give my explicit consent, you may assume ownership of my feline companion.

You exude a delightful aroma, leading me to ponder if your taste is equally pleasing. (Feel free to gently nibble or caress his body after uttering these words.)

I trust that you possess an affinity for playful taunting, as my intention is to engage in such acts until you reach the precipice of overwhelming anticipation.

It brings me immense joy when you cast your gaze upon me in such a manner.

I intend to elicit vocal expressions of pleasure from you, but only when I am fully prepared to do so (deliver this statement while maintaining eye contact and engaging in intimate stimulation).

Please sense the level of moisture that you have elicited (Extend your hand and guide him to place it upon your genital area to perceive the wetness you have experienced).

Please take a seat and remove the zipper on your trousers. You're mine now.

Please make your way to the bed and kindly shut your eyes. I intend to claim you as my own.

I anticipate your preparedness, as the desire for intimacy between us has been present throughout the day. Now that my longing is fulfilled, I intend to wholeheartedly partake in the experience.

What actions do you intend to take towards me? (Please express this sentiment in a reserved manner and use gentle eye contact, he will greatly appreciate it!)

How may I be of assistance to you? (Utter this phrase as you unzip his trousers, prior to making contact with his genitals.)

I derive great pleasure whenever you bestow upon me such affectionate kisses. (Express this sentiment when he is engaging in intimate acts on the areas that bring you pleasure.) This approach subtly directs him towards your preferences.

I love your cock.

I can perceive your presence with such intensity that it is as if I can literally taste you. (Phrase this as you caress and bestow gentle affection upon his abdominal region and upper legs.)"

You have an exquisite flavor, my darling.

I have a deep affection for providing oral pleasure to you.

Experiencing the flavor of your appendage instills within me an intense desire to engage in vigorous intimate activity with you.

I desire for you to ejaculate onto my facial region, my beloved.

Kneel down and engage in oral stimulation of my vagina. Now. I request you to assume an open stance and engage in self-touch while expressing the following statement.

Do you desire to savor the intimate essence of my personhood, my dear? Observe the impact you are having on my well-being. (Please utter these words while engaging in self-stimulation.) This drives men wild!)

I experience a sense of moral depravity when in your presence. I simply desire to engage in oral relations with your phallus.

I desire for you to engage in an intense intimate experience with me. Make me scream.

I am desperately in need of your presence within me.

Please convey your level of desire for this opportunity.

Mmmm, good boy. Please increase or decrease the pace at which you are performing oral stimulation. (Use this to communicate your desired rhythm or pace to guide him during oral pleasure.)

You appear exceptionally attractive at this moment. (Utter this phrase when he is actively engaged in performing oral sex on you). He will become enthusiastic and desire to engage in it further!

I would appreciate it if you could grasp my hair gently and engage in oral intimacy.

I desire to orally pleasure you.

Please subject me to deep throat stimulation with that erect phallus.

Engaging in oral pleasure with you greatly arouses me.

I am willing to undertake any action necessary to experience your intimate presence, my dear. Kindly instruct me on the tasks you wish for me to undertake.

Are you attracted to my feline companion, my dear? I derive pleasure from your acts of sexual stimulation towards me.

Oh, darling, please engage in intimate relations with me. Please, baby. I need it now. I have a strong desire for you. I kindly request that you please provide me with this.

This is my property, and I have the right to exercise autonomy over it as I see fit. "(Express this when you are prepared to engage in oral stimulation on his genital.)

I am currently experiencing a significant level of financial constraint. I am eagerly anticipating the intimate connection we will share.

I am the sole individual who engages in sexual activity with this rooster, do you comprehend me? Please hand it over, and express your message assertively.

You shall refrain from producing any auditory expressions unless I explicitly permit you to do so. Please recline and maintain silence, exhibiting good

13

behavior akin to that of a well-mannered child. (Say this when engaged in oral intimacy and he is expressing audible pleasure.)

DISRUPTING UNFAVORABLE SEXUAL COMMUNICATION

In order to optimize your child's receptiveness and ascertain your role as the primary authority on matters of sexual education, it is imperative to maintain a commitment to sincerity whilst imparting knowledge about sex and sexuality to your child. To varying extents, each one of us assumes a role as educators in matters pertaining to sexual behavior.

It is imperative for us, as parents, to demonstrate honesty in our guidance for our children, just as the educators I mentor to teach sex education are required to exhibit honesty in their instruction for their students.

Consequently, we are obligated to expose our children to authentic environments in order to impart knowledge to them.

Technique for traversing the road by visually scanning in both directions

Consider the manner in which you instructed (or intend to instruct) your child on the proper procedure for safely navigating a road crossing.

Namely, you will engage in numerous discussions concerning the act of crossing at the designated intersection, ensuring to visually inspect all directions before proceeding onto the road, and adhering to traffic signals during your crossing. You will perform various scripted simulations that mimic potential situations she could encounter while crossing the street, emulating real-life incidents.

As an illustration, a driver could disregard a red traffic signal, or find themselves at a sizable intersection where numerous vehicles intend to make turns simultaneously, or even arrive at an intersection that lacks traffic lights and features only stop signs. In order to ensure your child's safety while crossing the road, you will carefully prepare for all possible situations that they might come across.

Additionally, you will accompany her in practical exercises of safely navigating street crossings. Upon doing so, you will partake in authentic pedagogy (refer to the sidebar) at its fundamental essence: instructing your child by affording her the opportunity to actively apply the concepts you desire her to comprehend.

What does it signify to instruct with genuineness?

Authentic pedagogy, commonly referred to as genuine instruction, is an educational approach aimed at faithfully recreating real-world scenarios to the greatest extent possible. Experiential learning constitutes an essential element of genuine pedagogy. If one is engaged in instructing an individual on the art of ascending a rock wall, it is advisable to encourage them to engage in practice sessions.

If you are instructing your child on pedestrian safety measures, you may engage in practical training exercises with him as well. Indeed, it is a fact that educating one's child about sexuality through real-life experiences presents a greater difficulty (as engaging in sexual activities with one's child is clearly not a viable option, is it?).

Nevertheless, there exist a range of approaches that can be employed to replicate real-life situations. In relation to the topics that will be addressed in this book, encompassing aspects such as sexual emotions, influences from peers, making decisions of a sexual nature, and understanding gender differences, I shall furnish you with tangible illustrations of effective techniques applied in real-life circumstances.

Discuss Your Perspectives on Sexuality and Personal Relationships

It is important to consistently express your personal values in relation to the topic you are instructing on. Our values influence our perspectives regarding morality, discerning the positive and negative, valuing what is precious, and abstaining from what is undesirable. As your children evolve their personal beliefs and principles, they will still rely on your guidance and instruction.

Suppose you wish to broach the subject of HIV/AIDS with your young child, who is five years old. The conference will address the ethical dimension of embracing and providing compassionate care to individuals living with HIV/AIDS, or those who face the challenges arising from a potentially life-threatening illness. It is advisable to inculcate in your child the virtue of providing aid to individuals who are ill or injured.

Might you be interested in engaging in a conversation regarding homosexuality with your five-year-old?

This presents an opportune moment to foster in your child a lasting disposition towards embracing and respecting individuals who identify as gay or lesbian.

It is disheartening if one fails to recognize the importance of accepting individuals irrespective of their sexual orientation. It is a tragic reality that every year, lives are lost in our nation due to the prejudice against individuals perceived as gay or lesbian. It is imperative that we eradicate this mindset permanently.

The capacity of a youth to cultivate tolerance is augmented through the engagement in general discussions pertaining to tolerance.

Engaging in conversations about homosexuality with your five-year-old child will not induce any homosexual tendencies, just as promoting tolerance towards individuals of different races will not alter your child's skin color.

How can one effectively communicate the concept of homosexuality to one's child in a respectful and impartial manner? You assert that, akin to the romantic entanglement between individuals of opposite genders, there exists a possibility for affection to arise between males and females. Two individuals of the same sex develop a deep affectionate bond.

Two women who engage in this behavior are homosexual women. Individuals who identify as homosexual can be classified under the aforementioned term. It is highly probable that a young child may exhibit disinterest at this juncture and respond with a simple acknowledgement before moving on. You may also include the fact that certain individuals hold unfavorable opinions towards individuals who identify as gay or lesbian. Certain individuals engage in actions that seek to inflict harm upon individuals who identify as gay or lesbian.

That, from my standpoint, is both alarming and incorrect. As one grows older, it is crucial to cultivate an attitude of appreciation towards individuals who identify as homosexual. It is worth considering that even a young child, aged five for instance, could potentially identify as homosexual. This realization underscores the significance of imparting values of acceptance and empathy. You desire for your offspring to embrace their own identity without reservations, irrespective of their sexual orientation.

Educate your child on the distinction between ethical and unethical behaviors.

When imparting to your children your beliefs regarding sexual values and orientations, you are simultaneously conveying your personal interpretation of what is deemed morally correct or objectionable. One cannot surpass the role of a responsible parent by engaging in consistent dialogue and unwaveringly upholding the boundaries related to sexuality that are expected from their child. When engaging in the aforementioned actions, you are precisely accomplishing the task at hand.

• When communicating with your six-year-old, who may have a habit of touching himself in public areas of your residence, you might say, "Engaging in self-touching is something that is permissible, but it should be done privately." Later, during a subsequent conversation, you could express, "It has been quite a while since you engaged in any masturbation in the living room, and that brings joy to Mommy."

• You convey to your eight-year-old child, "I have concerns when you use the expression 'That's so gay' as it may be perceived as offensive towards individuals identifying as gay." Subsequently, a few days later, you express, "I've observed that recently you have refrained from using the word gay in a manner that troubles me." "I hold great affection for you."

• You communicate to your ten-year-old, "I believe it is inappropriate for anyone to engage in sexual activity until they reach adulthood and experience genuine love," and as time passes, "I consistently admire your choice to postpone engaging in intimate relations until reaching a mature age."

• You express to your ten-year-old fifth-grader, "In my honest opinion, I believe you still lack the maturity required to engage in romantic relationships at your age. However, I am glad to see that you haven't pursued a romantic relationship thus far." It is crucial for us as parents to communicate our stance on appropriate and inappropriate behavior regarding sexual subjects to our children.

What is the underlying cause of our reluctance to take action? A significant number of parents who participate in my school seminars exhibit a reluctance to establish appropriate boundaries regarding sexuality for their children. Some individuals have openly acknowledged engaging in sexual activity during their childhood, without experiencing any negative repercussions. This prompts the question, why are we imposing such severe punishments on our young ones?

A mother exclaimed. Has the father recently inquired about whether he should inform his daughter that she won't engage in sexual activity until she experiences romantic love? Why? I refrained from speaking.

It is incumbent upon us, as parents, to establish boundaries. Our next task is to determine and discuss those boundaries in a manner that fosters attentiveness from our children. We eagerly anticipate undertaking this endeavor once more within the context of middle school. Based on our analysis, it is projected that approximately 7% to 10% of children in the United States will engage in sexual activity prior to reaching the age of thirteen. Approximately five to seven and a half million children are expected to engage in sexual behavior prior to reaching adolescence.

I express my affection towards you and wish to convey an important message that aligns with my love for you. It is my sincere hope that you refrain from engaging in sexual activity until reaching adulthood, and even then, only engaging in such relationships with an individual whom you hold in high regard, trust, and genuinely love. I comprehend that receiving this information may prove challenging, yet it is of utmost importance for you to comprehend our parental beliefs regarding the appropriate timing for engaging in sexual relations.

While it may seem as though your child is incapable of tolerating the idea, given their tender age, you could respond by saying, "I acknowledge that this might be challenging to accept, but please believe me when I emphasize the importance of comprehending your parents' words." And in the present moment, perceiving it is more desirable than at a future juncture, when the opportunity might have passed. We will continue to engage in similar discussions as you mature and gain more life experience." "Several high school students have expressed to me, Dr. Michelle, that they didn't fully grasp the significance of the information you shared with them during their fifth-grade years.

Our children must possess knowledge about subjects such as self-pleasure, same-sex relationships, birth control, termination of pregnancy, oral sexual activity, adult intimacy aids, appropriate dress lengths, and pants worn below the waistline, among other relevant matters.

It is crucial that we proactively communicate our viewpoints to our children prior to them developing their own perspectives on these matters. It is highly improbable for you to experience any sense of shame. Allow us to consider a hypothetical scenario where you hold the following perspective:

• Self-stimulation is deemed permissible as long as it is performed in a discreet and private manner.

• Engaging in oral sexual activity is considered acceptable within the context of mutually caring and devoted relationships; however, it is important to acknowledge that it carries the risk of contracting HIV and other infectious diseases, as it falls under the category of sexual intercourse.

• In the event that a young woman chooses to dress in attire that exudes sensuality, heterosexual adolescent males may be inclined to interpret this as an indication of her desire for engaging in intimate activities, consequently sparking a reciprocal interest in partaking in such actions.

• Despite the effectiveness of condoms as the sole contraceptive method to prevent HIV transmission, abstinence remains the most favorable choice.

• While the act of abortion is indeed regrettable, it is imperative that it be granted legal authorization.

By the age of 10, these values statements can be imparted to your child. What is your perception or stance on the matters at hand? What are your most valuable assets? We\'ll cover a wide range of topics as we progress through this book together.

Form a Bond

I am uncertain if I can adequately emphasize the significance of connection.

Arguably, the paramount element in a child's existence lies in the establishment of a nurturing, respectful, and reliable bond with a significant adult over an extended period. Whom could be more suitable to assume this role than Mom or Dad, or another entrusted individual? A significant portion of the topics that have been addressed thus far in this chapter can assist us in fostering stronger connections with our children.

Fostering a deep connection with our children encompasses far more than simply cultivating a friendship, engaging in activities together, spending leisurely time with them, or having expectations of them complying with our requests. Bonding entails a substantial, profound, enduring, and mutually beneficial connection with another individual, in this particular case, your offspring.

Fostering a deep connection with your child establishes a safeguard that shields them from the formidable challenges prevalent in today's youth-centric environment. Establishing a strong emotional connection with your child greatly reduces the likelihood of their involvement in substance abuse, violent behavior, or risky sexual activities.

That is indeed correct: by consciously dedicating time to be with your children, you will enhance the probability of them abstaining from participating in these detrimental activities. A considerable portion of the information I just presented can be applied in this context. We possess significant capability to influence our children's sexual conduct in a constructive manner.

Cleavage

Exhibiting the décolletage can be regarded as a provocative gesture that holds significant allure for a considerable number of gentlemen. If employed judiciously, you will possess the ability to allure him at your discretion.

Presented here are a selection of alluring images that may be of interest to you:

Please capture a conventional shot showcasing the individual's décolletage. Ensure that you capture it from a vertically inclined perspective to enhance his visual experience.

Please capture an image while wearing only your brassiere. He will lose his sanity! Upon delivering the image, transmit to him this correspondence: 'I require assistance in removing this...'

This particular item has been widely acclaimed by a considerable number of gentlemen. I have engaged in conversations with numerous young ladies who have expressed their unanimous admiration for it. Please disrobe entirely and then capture an image of your breasts while ensuring that your fingertips conceal the nipples. It is an exceedingly unkind form of provocation that ought to be deemed as a punishable offense!

Once you have forwarded a selection of these captivating photographs, consider relaying the following messages to him: "

I derive immense pleasure from the sensation you provide when you lightly apply suction to my nipples.

I am experiencing heightened sensitivity in my nipples due to my attraction towards you.

I greatly appreciate the pleasure derived from your stimulation of my breasts.

I am eagerly anticipating your arrival at my residence...

A highly recommended short video to share with your significant other involves cheerful, rhythmic movements resulting in lively bosom dynamics. A brief duration of approximately four or five seconds will be adequate. Express a slight degree of discontent as well. Once you dispatch such a message, his ability to focus on other matters will be greatly diminished for the duration of the day.

Shower/Bath

Are you planning to engage in personal hygiene through bathing or showering? It presents an excellent occasion to capture alluring photographs for your significant other.

Utilize these images to subtly arouse his interest and evoke an immediate sense of desire.

Capture an image of yourself in the mirror while wearing a loosely draped towel around your body, ensuring that your chest is only partially exposed.

Please capture an image of your lower limbs and/or feet amidst a bubble-filled bath.

Indulge in a bath and adorn your décolletage with a foamy veil. Next, take an alluring photograph for him, ensuring that your nipples remain concealed.

Provide him with these explicit messages after sharing those provocative photos with him: "

I fervently desire a passionate encounter in the shower.

After my completion, you shall also require a shower.

The sensation of this water against my skin is truly delightful. However, the sensation derived from your genitalia is consistently more pleasurable.

To playfully provoke him, lightly immerse your feet in the water in a brief video clip. Wouldn't you desire to be present alongside me?

Bikini

Going to the beach? Before you depart, consider capturing some attractive images for your partner. Residing in close proximity to the beach, I am aware of the strong attraction men have towards viewing women in swimsuits.

"Here are several compelling suggestions:

Enlist the assistance of a female companion to capture a tasteful, full-body photograph of yourself in an appealing swimwear ensemble.

Capture an aesthetically pleasing photograph highlighting the neckline and décolletage area.

Capture an image of your swimwear bottoms. If his preference lies with the posterior, it will greatly agitate him.

Here is an alternative way to express the same idea in a more formal tone: "Allow me to provide you with a suitable text message to send him following the transmission of those provocative images:"

I long for your presence so you could help me remove my swimwear.

Could you kindly provide your opinion on my attire?

Would you be interested in partaking in a swimming activity?

To add allure to the video, gracefully spin before the camera whilst donning a bikini as a stylish gesture for him. Subsequently, message him with the following announcement: "I am patiently anticipating your arrival..."

Ass

If your partner has a preference for the buttocks, do not hesitate to indulge him. Share tantalizing images of your alluring rear and witness his anticipation until your next encounter.

Allow me to present to you a selection of concepts:

Capture an image of your buttocks by utilizing a mirror. Don\\\'t over-think it. Upon catching sight of your posterior, he will instantaneously succumb to your influence, akin to malleable clay in your grasp.

Please capture an image while wearing a thong. Thong undergarments exude an exceptionally seductive appeal.

If you are experiencing a sense of impurity, consider forwarding these two brief videos to your significant other:

Gently caress your posterior region and emit a sensuous vocalization. The duration of the video should be restricted to a maximum of two or three seconds. In a formal tone, you could convey the same message as follows: "Subsequently, send him the following message: 'I have behaved inappropriately.'" I believe it would be beneficial for you to administer corporal punishment upon your return home. Such an action is likely to greatly heighten his interest and enthusiasm.

If you happen to be in the company of a friend, kindly request her assistance in performing a task wherein she attempts to dislodge a coin from the posterior region of your physique, under the assumption that you have diligently engaged in squat exercises to maintain the muscular strength and tone of said area. Men absolutely love this. Indeed, my companion had an intense reaction to this latest video.

Things Not To Say

It would be regrettable if we failed to allocate a portion of our discussion to address inappropriate conversational topics. We will provide guidance to help you avoid potential obstacles, as the possibility exists for both significant errors and significant successes. It is important to bear in mind that the primary objective of engaging in dirty talk is to evoke a provocative and sensual mental imagery in both your and your partner's thoughts. Objects that do not conform to the appealing structure or

Being excessively distant from being hot will inevitably hinder the course of events, just as anything that could induce discomfort.

Don't:

1. When reference is made to an infant.

Those hips are conducive to childbearing. Hold on... what? I highly appreciate the desire to enter into matrimony and commence a family, however, the essence of sexual intimacy lies in fostering immediate emotional connection with one's partner, irrespective of the stage of the relationship. The sole conceivable deviation would be if you and your partner are actively engaged in endeavors aimed at conceiving a child. Nonetheless, the usage of the term "baby" typically connotes obligations, dedication, and an assortment of weighty matters that one may prefer not to delve into during moments of intimacy. It is advisable to avoid discussing infants within the confines of the bedroom.

2. Mention the former partner or the parents!

It is advised not to bring up the topic of your previous romantic partner, even if your intention is to compare their physical appearance with your current partner. Furthermore, when engaging in sexual activities, it is crucial to prioritize the present moment and abstain from discussing potentially sensitive matters. It is highly advisable to refrain from introducing any topics that may cause discomfort or unease during intimate relations. Your act of lavishing me with praise and attention surpasses all expectations. However, it will undoubtedly lead to an immediate cessation of your desired outcomes.

The parents are an additional topic that should not be discussed. Who desires recalling individuals whilst engaging in intimate acts? Do you recall the sequence in Seinfeld referred to as 'the undergarments that your mother arranged for you?'

3. Exhibit a polite and pleasant disposition

Dirty entails a slight exploration of boundaries, hence the concept of 'making love' appears overly innocent and juvenile. Does the expression "I desire to engage in passionate intimacy with you until you vocalize pleasure" pique your interest? Indulging in an enchanting soirée accompanied by fine wine, effervescent elixirs, and the soft glow of flickering candles provides a captivating ambiance conducive to igniting passion. However, the introduction of explicitly provocative discourse extinguishes the flame of romance. The allure of provocative conversation lies in its subtly daring essence; thus, it is advisable to adopt a mischievous demeanor rather than a polite one.

4.Puns

Puns can be a source of amusement, yet it is advisable to refrain from incorporating them within the confines of the bedroom. They undermine the ambience that you have diligently orchestrated, inciting your partner's uncertainty and impulsiveness. "You are like an apple that requires me to peel away its layers," may seem alluring and intriguing, but it also appears somewhat...peculiar. With regard to engaging in provocative language, opt for a straightforward approach and demonstrate your cleverness in contexts beyond the confines of the bedroom.

5.Parrot

It is conceivable that your partner has expressed something of great allure, prompting your desire to reciprocate with a gesture equally captivating. Rather than merely acknowledging or echoing their statement, contemplate an alternative response. Engaging in explicit conversation involves a reciprocal dynamic, characterized by mutual participation and interaction. If you genuinely desire to reiterate their words, consider introducing some variation.

Individual of unfavorable influence: I strongly aspire to exert great pressure upon you.

Woman: I desire to be vigorously engaged with you.

I desire greatly to exert my dominance over you.

Woman: I desire for you to engage in vigorous activity with me, similar to the forceful pounding of a jackhammer.

Incorporate the Topic of Food into the Conversation

Food should not be incorporated into explicit language, unless it is used in the context of an intimate food fight, feeding one's partner in a seductive manner, or sensually enjoying a delectable treat off of one's partner's body. Complimentary comparisons involving hot toast may elicit laughter, yet there is a possibility that it could disrupt the flow or progress of the conversation. Could you please clarify whether there is any merit to the assertion that uttering the phrase, 'Your zucchini possesses such considerable length and firmness,' yields any tangible benefits for individuals?

7. Allude to Non-Related Areas of the Anatomy 7. Make Reference to Unassociated Regions of the Human Body 7. Mention Areas of the Anatomy Not Directly Related

Observe my well-developed physique, as my muscles are prepared to exert maximum effort in order to ensure your satisfaction and comfort. Does this statement not strike you as peculiar? Refrain from seeking to include elements in a provocative image that do not naturally belong. Please remember that your objective is not to produce a workout video, but rather to create an appealing image.

8. Discuss bodily fluids of a non-sexual nature.

Certain individuals may exhibit a preference or inclination towards engaging in practices involving the exchange of bodily fluids such as urine or blood. However, it is advisable to limit one's exploration to those fluids strictly associated with sexual activities, namely saliva, semen, and vaginal secretions. It is imperative to avoid provoking any disruption or disturbance to the atmosphere or occasion, as it may give rise to the misconception that you possess an overwhelming presence that is difficult to manage.

9.Critique

While it may appear evident, it is imperative to exercise heightened sensitivity when engaging in explicit conversations to mitigate the risk of any unintentional misinterpretations of your words.

In consideration of the interpersonal dynamics at play, an unintended expression that does not arise from a critical intent may potentially be misconstrued as such, particularly when it pertains to a subject matter that deeply resonates with one's partner. When expressing the sentiments of urgency or insufficiency, please exercise caution regarding your vocal delivery. Rather than adopting a bossy or critical approach, one can appeal to the other person in a captivating manner.

10. The phrase 'You can if you want' exhibits a lack of decisiveness.

Despite its outward appearance of politeness, it in fact elicits aversion. Your associate has recklessly exposed themselves to potential harm, and they have made an inquiry regarding their ability to engage in a particular activity ... They require your assertiveness or guidance in some form.

It could have a disconcerting effect and potentially disrupt the atmosphere if you choose not to provide them with a definite response. Exhibiting assertiveness and clearly articulating one's desires is equally alluring. Ensure that there is clarity regarding your desires, requirements, and aspirations concerning both yourself and your partner. Please indicate your enthusiastic affirmation by responding with a resounding "YES!!" if you possess an affinity for it. In a more formal tone: "Provide guidance by delicately expressing, 'Perhaps tonight is not the appropriate time, my dear. Might I suggest an alternative option?'"

11. Exaggerating the Situation

The concept of Dirty Talk revolves around creating an imagery that allows for shared enjoyment and sustained focus on the present experience. It can be enjoyable to create an enticing environment for your romantic partner, but caution must be exercised to prevent venturing into a realm where individuals possess dual heads and five breasts, which may surpass the boundaries of one's imagination. Ultimately, it will elicit negative emotions in all individuals involved.

12.Be TOO Freaky

As an extension of the previous two "prohibitions," refrain from displaying an exaggerated level of peculiarity in general. Although the primary objective of engaging in explicit communication is to explore boundaries and test limits, it is crucial to recognize that there are inherent boundaries. The discussion prior to engaging in sexual activity is of utmost importance. It is imperative to show respect towards your partner's boundaries and collectively establish a comfortable environment.

Mistakes to Avoid

What are the common mistakes I should steer clear of when engaging in defamatory speech?

Do not excessively fixate on matters of size.

Do not excessively fixate on bodily proportions, be it pertaining to thighs, breasts, genitalia, or any other specific feature. It can be quite challenging to execute this correctly. Moreover, it is possible that you may unintentionally trigger your partner's vulnerabilities. Although you may have an appreciation for your lady's petite bosom, it is important to consider that she may feel uncomfortable or self-conscious when you unintentionally emphasize her lack of breast size. Furthermore, refrain from referring to a gentleman's phallus as "humongous" knowing well that it is merely of standard dimensions. Taking note of the gentle prominence of her nipples or expressing admiration towards his firm arousal would be more suitable choices.

If you have no intention of fulfilling the delivery of the goods, please refrain from making such statements.

If one were to make statements such as, 'You have exhibited improper behavior, young lady or gentleman.' I shall impose disciplinary measures upon you. Therefore, it is imperative that you ensure full compliance. Additionally, it is crucial to communicate your unwavering commitment to fulfill your commitments to your partner. Alternatively, in the absence of such conditions, all of that dubious discourse bears no consequence.

Exercise caution in avoiding the dissemination of misguided optimism within the cognitive sphere of your romantic partner. Unless you possess the proficiency to thoroughly examine an alternative anomaly, refrain from alluding to its likelihood.

One should refrain from committing sensual phrases to memory.

It is more advisable to devise one's own utterances rather than resorting to researching a multitude of derogatory terms employed by others. A meticulously prepared environment exudes an undeniable allure. It is important to consider that nobody else in this world truly understands the intricacies and desires of your ideal romantic partner.

Refrain from employing questionable language to elicit compliments.

That is except if you\'re available to the chance of dissatisfaction. When you express curiosity about your romantic partner, such as by inquiring, "Did you appreciate the manner in which I employed my oral skills?" your intention is not self-centered, but rather focused on seeking their thoughts and feelings. Moreover, seeking validation through soliciting compliments reveals a profoundly unappealing insufficiency of self-assurance.

Do not succumb to the tendency of expressing phrases such as, 'Oh yes, that sensation is pleasurable.' It tends to quickly lose its relevance. It conveys an air of indolence, automatism, and even absence of genuineness. It is imperative to provide greater precision and elaboration, as previously stated. Devote full attention to your partner's actions. As a result of this, their affection towards you will be further amplified. For example, it was remarkable how you adeptly manipulated your tongue along my organ and performed that skilled maneuver.

Disparaging comments like "Oh yes, indulge in my intimate regions!" exhibit characteristics reminiscent of explicit and degrading adult content. Using explicit language from pornography can be perceived as a derogatory act towards the intelligence of your romantic partner. It is undesirable for your ideal partner in the realm of intimacy to hold the belief that you are assuming their identity. Rather than enhancing it, it compromises its integrity. Your romantic partner will undoubtedly begin to doubt their own capabilities, thus leading us to our subsequent negative aspect.

Do not engage in any endeavors to simulate or fabricate an orgasm.

Upon experiencing this, your romantic partner may begin to question the authenticity of previous intense climaxes they have encountered. It is advisable to refrain from expressing phrases like, "You make me sexually aroused," to your romantic partner, even if it may appear to be alluring. It is essential to maintain sincerity in relationships as attempts to deceive are often perceivable by the other person involved. Remember to giggle.

Excessive tension may lead to difficulty in articulation. Couples in contented partnerships understand the significance of sharing laughter together as opposed to directing it towards each other. Be ready to encounter a handful of obstacles and address them with a touch of levity.

Strategies For Establishing A Romantic Connection With A Woman

Indications that she is attracted to you

A lady possesses an inherent enigma, and the greater the endeavor to unravel her concealed gestures, the more intricate matters tend to evolve. To expedite the more challenging aspects of courting a woman, it is essential to acquire the skill of interpreting her nonverbal cues. By discerning the true intentions behind her actions, even when unspoken, you will undoubtedly attract her attention more effectively than others. Presented below are five discernible indications that she may have a heightened interest in pursuing a physical encounter with you this evening. Utilize these cues to determine her inclination towards an intimate engagement.

She is initiating the advances towards you. She engages in flirtation to some extent, but there is a noticeable distinction when a lady is actively reciprocating your advances. Attempt to deduce the answer by observing her behavior. It appears as though she is eagerly anticipating your initiation of action. She is attempting to provide indications regarding what she wishes to communicate to you, yet she is unable to articulate it explicitly. Hey, what more could be desired!!! The only requirement is to ensure optimal conditions for the satisfaction of both parties involved.

She is in a heightened state of emotion. One could argue that when humor is employed, she emits audible laughter or expresses her thoughts assertively. If it is evident that her mood noticeably improves in your presence, it signifies that your company elicits positive emotions within her.

Her proximity exceeds acceptable levels of comfort. She extends her hand toward you, making fleeting yet consistent contact. A woman who is aroused will endeavor to initiate a degree of intimacy and carefully observe your response. It is essential to carefully observe her nonverbal cues to determine her level of interest in engaging in activities later this evening.

She engages in playful banter and exhibits a teasing demeanor. It is as if she desires to embrace you, but she expresses it in a different manner, expecting you to reciprocate in the exact same manner! It becomes evident when a woman's intentions shift from mere flirting to something more provocative - when she becomes restless and excited, she may have a desire to retire to bed sooner than anticipated.

She demonstrates her interest. One can ascertain it through her responses to the information provided. When she poses numerous inquiries, she demonstrates a moderate level of curiosity and a genuine desire to gain a deeper understanding of your character. If an individual does not hold a favorable opinion of you, there is little reason to exert one's efforts, correct? If she regularly inquires about your well-being and expresses a desire to spend a significant amount of time together, or if she reschedules some of her commitments specifically to accommodate your presence, it is evident that she holds a sincere interest in you.

How to initiate a dialogue of a sensual nature with a female without appearing uncomfortable or unsettling
The objective at hand is to establish an undercurrent of sensual anticipation and cultivate a magnetic appeal towards her.
The reality is that if you continue to engage in casual conversations with a girl whom you find intriguing, she will naturally classify you as a friend within her perception.
She will perceive you solely as a platonic acquaintance, without experiencing any form of sexual attraction towards you.
The downside to this is that women or girls are aware of men's desire for sexual

intimacy with them. Any tentative proposal or overtures on your part can potentially trigger a woman to heighten her defenses.

Could you please explain the process to me? What is an appropriate approach to initiating a discussion of a sexual nature with a female without eliciting any concerns or objections?

In accordance with the aforementioned title, this article aims to provide guidance on initiating a conversation of a sexual nature with a female individual without evoking discomfort or unease.

You will acquire knowledge of the top three techniques for initiating a conversation about the subject of sex without overtly indicating your level of interest.

Before You Begin...

Please be aware that women tend to engage in discussions regarding intimate matters...

However, the majority of individuals exhibit hesitancy in discussing this matter with men whom they lack a sense of comfort or emotional bond with.

Prior to broaching sexual subjects with a woman or girl, it is essential to establish a meaningful connection with her.

It would be more advantageous if she is displaying some indications of interest. As an example, these actions could be observed when she is tending to her hair, making physical contact with you, or moving in closer during conversations.

Having acknowledged that, let us proceed... Regarding the initiation of a dialogue of a sexual nature with a female.

Here is a guide on initiating a dialogue of a romantic nature with a female individual:

Recommendation #1: Discuss matters from a sexual standpoint.

Suppose you are discussing a film.

Please refrain from expressing your admiration for the car chase sequence and the protagonist's physicality in the movie to her.

Conversely, elucidate the notion of your admiration for the amorous bond depicted among the characters.

And your appreciation for the sensuality portrayed in their scenes. Subsequently, you inquire whether there are alternative films that have had a comparable influence on her, and subsequently prompt her to expound upon the reasons behind said impact.

Tip #2: Nourish her intellect

Incorporate mildly suggestive language or phrases into your everyday conversation with her.

One effective approach to accomplish this objective is through the utilization of sexual innuendos or double entendres. This refers to uttering a statement that may initially appear innocent, but holds the potential to be interpreted as indecent or sexual.

For instance:

This particular task or activity is quite challenging.

"Regrettably, I did not accompany her." (When discussing the party you attended.)

He came dangerously close to colliding with her vehicle.

Another effective method to stimulate her intellect or gradually introduce discussions of a sexual nature is to employ "That is what she said jokes" and "That is what he said jokes."

When she makes a statement such as:

Please place it within.

It is greatly enhanced when it is moist.

"Would you like to enter the premises?" (when she is extending an invitation for you to come into her apartment)

Afterwards, you reply by stating:

That is precisely what she uttered.

Alternatively, when she articulates something along the lines of...

You are rendering it challenging for me.

It is becoming increasingly challenging.

I desire to consume the entire item.

In that case, you may reply by stating: "

That is the statement that he made.

When she deliberately utters something suggestive, subsequently playfully taunt her for possessing a lascivious inclination.

Naturally, you would not desire to venture into this realm during the initial phases or when you have recently made acquaintance.

Initiate a conversation on an initial and superficial level, gradually progressing towards a more intimate and explicit discourse.

Once again, ensure that you have established a positive rapport with her beforehand. Subsequently, you commence incorporating vocabulary that contains sexual connotations into your discourse.

As time passes, he will become at ease discussing sexual subjects with you.

If she does not comply, it is likely that she is not yet at ease in your presence.

Upcoming, we will be discussing the art of initiating a conversation of intimate nature with a female...

Tip #3: Discuss a personal anecdote involving a friend that involves a romantic relationship.

For instance:

You may inform her that you have a female acquaintance expressing concerns about her boyfriend's reluctance to engage in oral intercourse.

She holds the belief that her partner harbors an aversion towards engaging in oral sex with her or is not discerning the hints he is being provided.

Now, inquire about how women can effectively propose such ideas to their male counterparts.

How do women suggest or imply such matters?

You are able to perceive the acts you are engaging in here... You are encouraging her to discuss sex in a focused manner.

If she engages in open conversation regarding the topic of sexuality, it can be inferred that she is at ease when discussing sexual situations with you.

Moving forward, she will commence engaging in conversations of a sexual nature with you.

In conclusion... How to initiate a conversation of a sensual nature with a female individual.

Comprehend this: Avoid discussing matters of a sexual nature with the girl or woman with whom you are engaging in conversation. Engage in discussions solely pertaining to the intimate aspects of others' lives.

Top Strategies to Enhance Your Sexual Confidence in Interactions with Women

Discover the Origin of Sexual Assurance

Sexual confidence arises from a deep understanding of how to bestow extraordinary pleasure upon a woman. It is the assurance that the woman accompanying you will have a unique and unforgettable experience. Having a comprehensive understanding of each stage, starting from the initial visual connection up until the final outcome, and possessing the ability to effectively cultivate a sense of eager expectation throughout the entire process. Commence by honing my method of progressing incrementally, followed by retreating periodically, and subsequently advancing more intensively, then retreating once more. The level of expectation and arousal that emerges from this situation will greatly distress her. Please be advised that I have previously issued a warning on this matter.

Break Free from the Mindset of Manipulation

Men are often intrigued by the methods to manipulate women into sexual encounters, specifically seeking knowledge of persuasive language or techniques. I am personally acquainted with several individuals who engage in this practice... Furthermore, I can assure you that it does not result in personal fulfillment. Refrain from adopting the approach of "manipulation mindset" and desist from attempting to ascertain the precise tactics needed to coerce a woman into complying with your wishes through dishonest means. It is highly advantageous to focus on cultivating one's persona as an engaging individual, adept at fostering genuine attraction in an authentic and ethical manner. Cease and desist any actions that evoke a sense of wrongdoing or ethical impropriety. There exist more favorable means to obtain your desires.

Cease the idealization of attractive female individuals

Many individuals are often deceived into assuming that if a woman possesses exceptional attractiveness, she is inherently truthful and unlikely to engage in actions such as stealing from or cheating on a person, or delivering false information. The fact remains that individuals can never possess complete moral perfection or absolute moral corruption. There exist circumstances in which ANY individual could resort to deception, cheating, theft, or disloyalty. Upon embracing the truth that individuals are inherently flawed and that even an aesthetically pleasing lady is, at her core, a human being, it becomes apparent that the woman for whom you harbor deep affection possesses an equal propensity for deceit and disloyalty as any other person. This realization should prompt you to remove her from the elevated position you have bestowed upon her. This constitutes a significant stride towards attaining a sense of sexual assurance.

What level of significance do physical appearance hold in terms of cultivating confidence within the realm of intimate experiences?

Physical appearance is not a determining factor in regard to one's level of sexual confidence.

One's physical appearance, age, height, weight, income, or personal preferences have no bearing on their ability to evoke emotions in a woman once an intimate connection has been established. It is noteworthy that once a woman has undergone an exhilarating intimate encounter with you, that singular experience will render all other matters inconsequential. It just won\\\'t matter. Envision yourself existing in this forthcoming era, which will aid in manifesting it as a self-fulfilling prophecy.

Postpone Your Gratification

Postponing the act of obtaining satisfaction becomes increasingly significant as one contemplates it further - and in the context of sexual experiences, it is undeniably essential. Not only does it enable the development of sexual tension and increase her desire for you, but the act of teasing and generating anticipation also serves as catalysts to enhance her arousal. In summary, the likelihood of arousing her and escalating the situation to a physical level is greater when you maintain a composed and collected demeanor. By relinquishing your desire for immediate outcomes, you will profoundly frustrate her.

Behave in a manner that treats sexual activity as customary.

Many men experience anxiety when it comes to engaging in sexual activity. They believe that they must alter their behavior when the moment arises. However, it is important to remember that sex is a natural activity, so it is best to maintain a sense of normalcy as things become more intimate. Do not excessively emphasize the matter; continue to enjoy yourself; persist in playful banter; maintain a lighthearted demeanor. Effortlessly and assuredly transition from one phase to another, while simultaneously deriving pleasure and maintaining an appearance of normalcy—because that is indeed the case.

Viewing Sex from a Different Perspective

Rather than emphasizing sex as the ultimate objective and focal point of your intentions, reframe it as merely one of your numerous goals. If you possess an affection for a woman and have made the conscious decision to allocate your time and exertion towards progressing in that direction, allow such an outcome to transpire organically. By removing the perceived significance of sexual activity and adopting a balanced perspective, one's relaxed demeanor can significantly increase their likelihood of experiencing it.

Overcome the Apprehension of Rejection

As you traverse each phase of a relationship with a lady - transitioning from a casual outing to engaging in physical affection such as touching and kissing, and subsequently further - the level of significance and potential consequences heighten progressively. Traditionally, males tend to experience heightened apprehension as they transition from one stage to the next, displaying diminished confidence when faced with increasingly intense circumstances. The apprehension does not arise from the prospect of being rejected or hindered, but rather from the alarming prospect of forfeiting all the progress that has been achieved and regressing completely. Fortunately, the greater level of involvement you attain, the higher the probability of your success. The subsequent phase encompasses reduced risk and enhances the likelihood of engaging in sexual activity. Remember this.

Analyzing Her Behaviors" or "Evaluating Her Conduct

If she halts your actions, it typically does not imply a complete cessation of her desire, but rather indicates that you have not succeeded in sufficiently arousing her. Please consider interpreting this phrase as "I am not currently prepared," instead of expressing the sentiment "Please leave, I no longer have affection for you." Cease your actions, recline, engage in casual conversation for a period of time, and simply unwind. Subsequently, intensify her arousal beyond its previous state. You are welcome to encourage her to initiate a request for sexual activity... or even beg. "Please" is a valuable term - instruct her in its usage and she will greatly appreciate your guidance.

Establish Contact with the Inner Animal

A lady desires a gentleman who is connected with his innate animalistic qualities. If he displays an excessive inclination towards logic, excessive analytical tendencies, excessive control, and excessive education, it indicates to a woman that he is incapable of embracing his primal instincts. At a primal level of understanding, a woman recognizes that this implies she will be unable to experience profound emotions towards him, and she is aware that he will be unable to generate any sexual sensations within her. Educate yourself, familiarize with, establish acquaintanceship with, and foster the inner creature within you. Acquiring knowledge in this domain is one of the most crucial steps you can take to elevate your level of sexual confidence.

The optimal strategy for engaging in intimate relations with a woman and fostering a deep desire within her for your companionship.

A strong, affectionate, and enduring partnership considers a vibrant sexual connection as an essential component. If one were to observe their surroundings, it would not be challenging to discern which couples genuinely exude happiness in their relationship. Behold the couples who maintain a passionate gaze towards each other! What enigmatic formula keeps their ardor aflame? It is highly likely that both individuals experience mutual sexual satisfaction within their relationship.

Many individuals are aware that women do not achieve orgasm with the same ease or speed as men. Many fail to comprehend that this approach merely contributes to the accumulation of sexual dissatisfaction, which is a prevalent issue among women. Sexual frustration can manifest in various detrimental ways within a relationship, culminating in a pivotal moment where both individuals face the sudden realization of the absence of passion, be it for one another or within their lives. By that time, even satibo capsules would prove ineffective in kindling the ardor.

It is fortunate that achieving female orgasm is not a challenging endeavor in reality. However, both individuals must exert effort towards this endeavor, which, upon reflection, adds an element of enjoyment to the process as well!

This step-by-step guide can be of assistance to you. It represents one of several resources devised by Gabrielle

Moore, a knowledgeable authority in the field of sexual education.

STEP 1

Partake in ample foreplay. Foreplay holds significant importance as it aids in inducing relaxation of her mind and directs her attention towards the impending act of lovemaking. It serves as a vital enhancer for female orgasm. It is also a means to foster connections, as numerous women view foreplay as a man's method of investing time and ensuring that sex encompasses more than just purely physical engagement but also revolves around intimacy.

Preparation for sexual activities can commence prior to the actual event, with anticipation building over a span of hours or even days. The extent of exploration in this regard is bound solely by one's imaginative capacities. As you maintain a heightened state of sexual tension, you will discover that it becomes more effortless to facilitate her orgasm once you engage in sexual intercourse.

STEP 2

If foreplay is considered a preliminary step, oral sex serves as the subsequent significant progression. Numerous women assert that oral sex is their solitary means of achieving orgasm. Therefore, if your objective is to ensure that she attains climax, it is advisable not to refrain from engaging in such activity.

When engaging in oral stimulation with your partner, it is advisable to approach it with patience rather than rushing. Demonstrate your deep affection for her by offering her your unwavering attention. Take pleasure in the journey as much as the destination, so to speak.

Initially, engage in gentle teasing and delicately apply your tongue. Once she directs her attention towards that particular area of her body, escalate the pace. When you observe an increase in her respiration rate and intensity, or detect tension in her legs, shift your focus towards her clitoris. Indulge in gentle circular motions encircling it with your tongue, followed by increased pressure and quicker licks.

In the event that she displays any signs of being highly aroused, it is imperative to adhere to the following guidance: Refrain from making any alterations to the current situation. Maintain the rhythm of your actions, and she will reach her climax in due course.

STEP 3

If your oral stimuli do not elicit an instantaneous orgasm in her, do not lose hope. Please remember that your fingers can also serve a beneficial purpose. Employ your index finger to gently trace the contours of her labia. Please exercise caution and apply a light touch to her. This is certain to invigorate her physique. Following that, proceed to bring your index and middle fingers into contact with one another, and subsequently trace circular motions around her clitoris.

Observe her physical demeanor closely, noting whether it displays signs of pleasure and relaxation or if it appears tense, akin to a taut string; this will provide insight into her level of arousal. Please do not neglect to pay attention to her expressions of discomfort and vocalizations.

One can employ the technique of alternating between the tongue and fingers to elicit stimulation of her clitoris. Similarly, if she communicates any indicators of heightened arousal, it is recommended to maintain the same approach. This method serves as an effective means to evoke intense pleasure and elicit vocal responses from her.

STEP 4

If clitoral stimulation has not yet elicited an orgasm, then consider attempting G-spot stimulation. Assuming that she is already aroused, gradually insert your index and middle fingers into her vagina, with the palm facing upwards. Upon entering, place your fingers in the "11 o'clock" position. Gently attempt to identify a slight elevation or swelling, resembling an engorged clitoris. Once you have located this position, congratulations... You have successfully discovered the elusive G-spot!

STEP 5

One can engage in various methods to activate the G-spot. One can make contact with it using their fingertips, trace leisurely or animated circles around it, or flick it vigorously resembling a rapid movement of a light switch. If desired, one could employ their thumb to provide stimulation to her clitoris in conjunction with stimulating her G-spot. This will undoubtedly provide her with a memorable orgasm.

Methods And Positions

Presently, we will delve into a comprehensive exploration of diverse Tantric sexual postures and methodologies that can be employed to enhance intimacy and enrich one's sexual relationship.

The Sidewinder: An Exploration

The present role is inspired by the Yoga pose with a corresponding name, affording an opportunity for profound penetration. Additionally, it enables the pair to maintain communication. In order to execute this technique, the woman ought to assume a lateral position and provide support to the weight of her upper body using her hands. She ought to elevate one of her legs and rest it upon her beloved's shoulder, while the other leg remains recumbent upon the bed. An alternative term for this equivalent position is "conversely, the male assumes a position behind the female and engages in penetration from the rear."

The Divine Union

The Yab Yum position is widely regarded as the most optimal scenario for engaging in tantric sexual practices. This activity is inherently straightforward to execute and allows for simultaneous climactic events. This role contributes to the animation of several locations. Similarly, at present, the gentleman possesses unoccupied hands, enabling him to caress his beloved's physique as he desires. Given that the couple would face each other, this allows for passionate embraces as well. The gentleman is expected to assume a seated position, with one leg over the other, preferably on the bed or a suitable surface, while maintaining an upright posture. The woman should position herself astride him, crossing her legs over his lower back. It considers intermittent developments that may be delayed but ultimately contribute to the couple's successful achievement of a well-planned culmination.

The Fastening Mechanism

This stance allows the gentleman to have a respectable view of his significant other's visage, and vice versa. This is a highly appealing position that enhances the pleasure experienced by both individuals involved. To execute this process, it is advisable to position the woman on an elevated platform, such as a table or even the kitchen counter. Afterwards, she will be required to lie back and use her hands to adjust the positioning of her upper middle and head by propping herself up on her elbows. The gentleman should maintain his position between her parted legs and proceed with penetration. This is a versatile demonstration which can extend beyond the confines of the room and is ideally suited for spontaneous engagement.

The Lepidopteran

This approach is widely acknowledged for facilitating a mutually profound state of pleasure in both individuals involved and accounts for thorough penetration. To execute this procedure, it is recommended that the young lady reclines upon the table, ensuring that her posterior rests at the edge thereof, while the man assists by gently elevating her lumbar region from the table surface. Subsequently, he should proceed to position both of her lower limbs atop his shoulders. He would have unrestricted access to her intimate area while positioned between her legs. Due to the positioning of her legs, the vaginal pathway is constricted, resulting in a snug fit. The gentleman should initiate penetration while her posterior is elevated in the air.

The Dual-Level Structure

This is an exceptionally evocative position that will aid in achieving a climax effortlessly. The gentleman will also be granted a proper view of all the activity transpiring below, while his hands will also have unrestricted opportunity to caress his partner's posterior. This role offers significant empowerment to women, as they possess full authority and influence within this domain. In order to execute this procedure, it is necessary for the gentleman to assume a seated position on the bed, with his legs bent and positioned beneath his body. The lady will then be required to face away from him and position her feet on either side of her beloved, ensuring that her feet are flat on the surface to provide her with some support. Once she has positioned herself on his erect penis, she may commence the motion by alternately moving forwards and backwards, or even opting for intermittent movements. The man should essentially relax and enjoy himself.

The least desirable location for anyone to find themselves in

This stance is indeed remarkable as it enables both parties to exert an equal level of control and intensity in order to achieve a highly satisfying sexual encounter. Individuals are currently in possession of an equal balance. In order to enact this scene, the gentleman is required to assume a seated position on the bed and brace his upper body with his knees. Afterwards, he will be required to retract the lower section of his legs and position them in a slightly spaced apart manner. The lady will subsequently be required to assume a comparable posture, but she will do so while constantly facing away from him. Her legs will be pressed against his scrotum, and her back will be firmly against his chest. Her lower extremities would be positioned together and subsequently placed in the void situated between his lower extremities, so that the man may engage in posterior penetration. For this situation to be persuading, it is essential for both partners to maintain close proximity to one another.

Skiff

This role entails a minor modification to the superior position held by the woman. Currently, it is advised that individuals position their bodies in a manner that allows both partners to maintain proper eye contact while engaged in the activity. To carry out this action, the gentleman should take a seat on a chair that has the ability to slightly recline. The woman will then need to sit on his lap and subsequently position her legs on either side of the seat. The young woman should independently initiate a comprehensive exercise regimen, or alternatively, her colleague may lend assistance by providing support beneath her posterior, facilitating coordinated vertical and horizontal movements.

The Aquatic Nymph

This is a variation of the butterfly stroke that exhibits slight variations, aiming to enhance comfort and grip. Currently, individuals have the capability to engage in an affectionate act of foot-pleasuring with their significant other. Please bear in mind that feet are commonly regarded as one of the most sensitive and erogenous areas of a woman's body. In order to execute this approach, the lady can anticipate a comparable scenario to that experienced during the butterfly position, with the distinction being the utilization of a cushion to provide support to her buttocks. Her legs should relax and be positioned at a 90-degree angle. The gentleman ought to position himself in close proximity to the table and clandestinely approach her.

Tsunami

This stance is highly pleasing and provides a sensory delight. This will leave you astounded. This stance exhibits a subtle modification of the distinguished ministerial manner. Currently, women should anticipate undertaking the tasks traditionally assumed by men in the field of teaching. In order to execute this action, the individual must assume a supine position, with his arms positioned closely to his sides. The woman should recline atop the man, while the man should insert his phallus into her vaginal cavity. The lady should properly relax her legs so that they are resting on his. It is advisable that her hands be placed on his forearm to offer her assistance. The woman will subsequently be required to initiate a motion of her pelvic area characterized by an upward and downward trajectory.

Lap Dance

This posture is an ideal position for a man to behold his beloved's physique in all its splendor. He will be granted the freedom to gently explore her physique, attending to her needs as necessary. The lady will avert her gaze from him in a manner analogous to if she were performing a lap dance for him. In order to carry out this demonstration, it is necessary for the gentleman to assume a seated position, ensuring that he maintains an upright posture. Subsequently, the woman will proceed to assume a seated position upon his thigh, finding equilibrium by resting her hands delicately upon his upper thighs or potentially his abdominal region. Subsequently, she will need to elevate herself gradually, positioning the posterior aspect of her lower legs, and slowly lower herself onto his phallus. An alternative interpretation of this scenario is when the woman lowers herself onto her partner's penis while maintaining direct eye contact. This intimate act grants him a favorable visual of her breasts. He has the option to intricately engage with and manipulate them for however long he deems fitting.

Pretzel

This represents yet another visually pleasing aspect that is also easily anticipated. This will result in the couple experiencing an overwhelming sense of attractiveness. To carry out this procedure, the couple should respectfully bow to each other. The gentleman ought to proceed forward, while the lady will cross her arms upon him. The woman will proceed to elevate herself and position her left leg adjacent to her beloved's right foot, ensuring that her foot is directed downwards. The gentleman will subsequently be required to position his left leg in proximity to her accurate foot. Upon observing a pair engaged in this position, they appear akin to a pretzel, one that exudes an enticing and appetizing allure.

The Dissemination

This is a critical and highly sought-after role. This affords the woman immense pleasure, as it enables her to caress her beloved and grants him the ability to bring her pleasure. To execute this protocol effectively, it is recommended for the woman to position herself discreetly at the periphery of the sofa or bed, ensuring that her legs are apart. The individual must proceed to position themselves centrally between her legs and penetrate her. She can approach him closely and engage in an intimate act of kissing while he gently explores her entire physique with his hands.

The Interweaving

This particular body position appears highly challenging and potentially difficult to replicate; nonetheless, with proper execution, it can be an immensely enjoyable experience. This posture exhibits a pleasing aesthetic appeal. In order to execute this plan effectively, it is recommended for the couple to position themselves in close proximity, facing one another. The gentleman is advised to position his legs on each side of his companion. The woman will subsequently be required to raise both of her legs and position them on either side of her beloved's torso, beneath his arms. The gentleman will support the lady's legs using his upper arms, and subsequently, the lady shall raise her own upper arms and position them upon his elbows. Subsequently, the gentleman will elevate his legs and carefully position them above her hands. This appears to be quite convoluted, wouldn't you agree? The considerable effort involved will justify the allocation of your time and energy.

The force of gravity

This could be considered among the most provocative tantric sexual offerings available. This is the epitome of all erotic gifts. The gentleman currently possesses complete supervision over his beloved, and both individuals involved will derive exceptional pleasure from this position. To enact this position, the woman should recline on her back upon the bed, while the man assumes a kneeling stance near her legs. Subsequently, he will proceed to gradually elevate her midsection from the bed, causing her head and shoulders to rest upon the bed while she maintains an asymmetric position. The gentleman has the choice to either position her legs at a 90-degree angle or penetrate her, alternatively, he can also separate them and position her feet just below his chest before entering her.

The Cascading Water Feature

In the present moment, it is advisable for the woman to place her hand upon her partner's phallus, proceeding to then gently and gradually allow her fingertips to make contact with his scrotum. It is advisable to apply a topical ointment to augment the level of comfort. Her hands ought to be positioned on both sides of his reproductive organs, and subsequently, she should carefully move her hands upward until they reach the sensitive tip of his penis. Once the task is completed, it is advisable for the woman to allow the man a period of relaxation before he proceeds to acknowledge the assistance he received. The gentleman is required to caress his partner's intimate area and explore all of her sensitive regions. He should gently caress her clitoral area and her labial region.

The Reptile

In this context, the woman should slowly elongate the shaft of her partner's genital organ by applying gentle pressure with one hand, while the other hand moves in small circular motions just below the tip. This can be likened to engaging in intricate and meticulous craftsmanship. Carry out these motions in a clockwise direction, and subsequently when you reach the tip of the penis, transition to an anticlockwise direction. Continue with this behavior for as long as your partner is able to tolerate it.

The Triangular Touch Technique in Tantric Practice

The woman should recline on her back with her legs slightly apart and flex them at the knee. The gentleman will subsequently be required to insert his index and middle fingers into her vaginal region and gently rotate them upwards, creating a motion commonly referred to as the "come here" technique. This will provide optimal stimulation for her G-Spot. This will elicit a delighted moan from her. While engaging in this action, he should place the palm of his other hand gently upon her lower midriff and administer a slight sensation of pleasure. This comprehensive provocation will expedite her descent towards a breaking point swiftly.

The Seesaw

This specific teeter-totter lacks any semblance of innocence. This is exceptionally suggestive. The woman is required to recline on her back upon the bed, ensuring that her pelvis is slightly positioned in an upward tilt. For this purpose, a cushion can be placed beneath her pelvic area. The gentleman will subsequently be required to elevate her feet and gently place them on top of each other so that her knees rest against her chest and the soles of her feet make contact with his chest. This position allows for unobstructed access to the female genitalia, ensuring that with an upward tilt, contact with the G-Spot is consistently achieved during each penetration.

Bathtub Entanglement

Have the gentleman recline in a filled bathtub, while the lady positions herself astride him with her back oriented towards him. Once penetration has occurred, he should assume an upright position, allowing both partners to face each other. Subsequently, she should cross her legs above him, and he should reciprocate in order to position their elbows beneath their partner's knees. Grasp each other tightly and initiate a reciprocating motion to exert an influential force. This permits the expression of fervent affection through intimate lip contact.

Romantic entanglement involving three individuals

The woman ought to lay supine on either the floor or the bed, subsequently elevating her left leg upwards. Her legs on the right side must be extended towards her right side, ensuring that both legs are positioned perpendicular to each other. Then, she will proceed to position her dominant hand and grasp her corresponding knee, creating a triangular shape on the bed utilizing her corresponding leg and hand. The man should slightly stoop and approach her, gently grasping her knee as he enters. This position would afford the individual enhanced pelvic control and additionally the opportunity to engage in tactile exploration from various perspectives, as desired. A subtle alteration can be introduced to this stance by instructing the gentleman to execute a circular motion with his hips while exerting pressure towards the lady; this maneuver will propel the couple towards their limit.

At this moment and in a state of tranquility

This position may serve as a means of momentarily alleviating the imminent climax. Tantric sexuality does not revolve around seeking rapid release, but rather emphasizes the indulgence in the profoundness of the experience. What could be a more fitting course of action than exercising self-restraint just prior to reaching the decisive moment. When you become aware of the potential for either yourself or your partner to reach climax, take a brief interlude to experience moments of respite and liberation from your current position. The gentleman has the ability to recline onto his side while maintaining his position within his companion simultaneously. This role merely entails capturing a brief interval of leisure. Gradual progression is acceptable, nevertheless, should you sense the imminent arrival of orgasm, it is advisable to momentarily cease, prolong the experience, and perhaps indulge in some intimate caresses and passionate kisses before resuming from where you left off. This particular position provides the essential physical proximity required to enhance the overall intimacy and well-being of the sexual encounter.

Intense Contest of Strength and Resilience

The lady is advised to assume a position with her legs crossed on the floor or another suitable surface. Subsequently, she should gradually lower herself onto his erect penis while also placing her legs around his back. This position will facilitate face-to-face interaction between the couple, allowing you to securely interlock elbows and lean in opposite directions for mutual support. This bears resemblance to engaging in a game of hesitant exchange. If both individuals display adaptability, one partner can incline their heads backwards and lean in a backward direction, distancing themselves from their counterpart. This role will consider the positioning of your bodies, leading to a close interaction with your partner. It establishes a strong connection and facilitates acceleration. Both partners have developed proficiency in playing the sport, consequently allowing the partners to exercise control over who enters.

The programming language Python

The gentleman should take a moment of repose at this time, ensuring that his legs are positioned in close proximity to one another, while his arms remain relaxed at his sides. The woman should lower herself onto his phallus and gradually establish a seated position. Once the man has entered her, she can elevate herself so as to lie fully on top of his body. Both of your physiques would be excellently attuned, enabling you to clasp each other's hands to accelerate and provide mutual support. The woman should proceed to gradually elevate her middle section from his, resembling a poised snake prepared to strike. She has the ability to exert pressure with her feet in order to facilitate further progress. You will both engage in close physical contact, with her breasts coming into contact with his chest, your hands grasped firmly, and his thighs brushing against hers. It factors in profound penetration, yet it also incorporates clitoral stimulation. Given that the couple will come face-to-face, this also encompasses engaging in passionate kissing. All the sensual areas of the body would be stimulated.

Ten Recommendations for Engaging in Conversations about Sexual Education and Personal Identity with Your Child.

1) Cultivate a sense of self-assurance and familiarity with the objective realities.

Individuals have varying levels of comfort when engaging in discourse related to matters pertaining to sexual well-being. It is acceptable for us to recognize that discussing matters of a sexual nature can be uncomfortable, provided that we also take responsibility for transmitting our unease.

The better you can cultivate a sense of self-confidence, the smoother the proceedings will become, and the more at ease your child will be when seeking your presence. Please be mindful that sex and sexuality encompass a broad spectrum of matters as well.

It is acceptable to shoulder responsibility for certain matters while entrusting other esteemed adults within your community, including professionals, to address issues that surpass your personal boundaries.

A means to enhance your level of comfort is by acquainting yourself with the pertinent information. It is imperative for children of a younger age to acquire fundamental knowledge. As they approach adolescence, it is crucial for them to be adequately prepared for the alterations they will experience in terms of physiological development, emotional responses, and burgeoning sexual sensations.

A multitude of reputable and precise sources exist, which can educate individuals in the art of providing developmentally suitable knowledge for youths of varying age groups.

Please bear in mind that there exist certain areas of expertise in which you possess proficiency that cannot be obtained through reading books. These assertions do not necessarily constitute "facts," yet they possess significant importance. Your values. Your community. Your child. Your life journey, encompassing both setbacks and triumphs.

Whilst maintaining a dialogue with your child is of utmost importance, it is equally crucial to cultivate self-awareness and understand what constitutes emotional well-being for oneself. If you have engaged in sexual encounters or made decisions in the past that you presently regret or find emotionally difficult to confront, please be aware that your conversations on this matter may become more intricate. Ensure your wellbeing by engaging in discussions pertaining to matters within your control. Bear in mind that you have the option of engaging individuals within your social network—such as co-parents, grandparents, or friends—to engage in open conversations with your child regarding topics that may prove challenging for you to discuss. Furthermore, there exist individuals of expertise in your child's sphere, such as educators, counselors, physicians, and healthcare practitioners, who possess extensive knowledge in these areas.

2) Initiate dialogue promptly and sustain an ongoing conversation.

It is imperative to initiate early discussions with our children and maintain open lines of communication continuously. It is imperative that even children in their early stages of development acquire knowledge regarding self-esteem, proper physical boundaries, and consideration for the emotions and boundaries of others.

When these subjects become integral to the core values that you regularly engage in conversations about, it will subsequently become more effortless to navigate these discussions as your children reach the stage of puberty and the onset of sexual emotions.

Typically, adolescents find it more convenient to engage in continuous dialogues regarding matters encompassing principles and security, as opposed to having sporadic discussions prompted by specific incidents. To put it differently, initiating a conversation prior to a first date or prom night would result in increased comfort for both parties involved - yourself and your adolescent - thereby fostering a higher level of receptivity.

Continuing dialogues engender an educational experience and may be esteemed as occasions to elucidate principles and deliberate on decision-making processes. Conversations held with a sense of urgency can give the impression of originating from a state of apprehension and may be construed as being overly authoritative or imperious.

Consequently, your well-intentioned efforts can have unintended negative consequences.

If you happen to be perusing this document prior to a forthcoming occurrence and lack the option of temporal reversal, it would be advisable to place significant emphasis on the underlying rationale for the ensuing discussion. Rather than imposing strict regulations, you are engaging in meaningful discussions regarding crucial subjects that will ensure their physical and emotional well-being.

3) Center the focus on core principles

There exist numerous educational resources where adolescents and young adults can acquire knowledge regarding the intricacies of sexual mechanics, puberty, and overall growth and maturation. These encompass educational modules on health, printed publications, and online resources. It is crucial that you ensure that your children acquire a strong foundation in understanding the principles surrounding wholesome sexuality from your guidance.

If you, along with other diligent adults, fail to engage in discourse on these subjects, the younger generation will inevitably internalize their principles from the vast array of media channels such as the internet, television, and music. In the eventuality of an unfavorable outcome, they will acquire knowledge from online pornography, potentially exposing themselves to damaging and disconcerting portrayals of sex and sexuality.

Additionally, they will acquire knowledge through interactions with their peers; however, these values, while potentially positive, may lack the depth and wisdom that comes with real-life encounters and challenges.

4) Foster an environment centered around reciprocal regard, encompassing deliberations on the preservation of well-being.

It is well understood that adolescents hold their parents' guidance in high regard and that parental knowledge plays a pivotal role in equipping young individuals with the necessary tools for a prosperous future. Furthermore, it is understood that adolescents tend to resist parental guidance when they perceive it as interfering with their personal affairs, but they appreciate it when it equips them with the knowledge and skills necessary to navigate the world securely and judiciously.

This knowledge is of pivotal importance in facilitating our discussions on matters concerning sex and sexuality – which undoubtedly pertain to deeply personal experiences. Hence, discussing individual relationships could potentially breach personal boundaries.

In a similar vein, inquiring about your adolescent's precise sexual conduct may encroach upon sensitive territory, potentially evoking a feeling of aversion.

Conversely, maintaining a general approach to conversations enables one to effectively engage in profoundly meaningful discussions with greater ease and comfort. Young individuals hold the belief that the responsibility of ensuring their safety lies with their parents, and numerous safety concerns form a significant aspect of our discourse on promoting healthy sexual conduct.

The preservation of emotional wellbeing is equally at risk. These emotional concerns encompass the art of "skillfully traversing through life." It is imperative that we deliberate upon the aspects of dignity for oneself and respect towards others. Boundaries and personal limits.

Attentively taking note of both verbal and non-verbal cues from others, in order to prevent engaging in actions that they do not wish for.

It is necessary to educate them in cultivating an appreciation for the inherent value of their bodies, ensuring their comprehension of their bodies' capabilities and promoting techniques to maintain their well-being.

5) Listen

Take heed of the perspectives and opinions of your adolescent children concerning matters pertaining to sexuality. The greater their trust in us, the better equipped we will be to steer them towards solutions that align with their developmental stage, particularly in relation to matters concerning sexuality. Active and attentive engagement with our teenagers is essential in fostering open communication with them. Occasionally, our brevity carries a greater impact, eliciting a more significant response from them.

Encourage them to talk. In the event that they pose an inquiry, inquire about their familiarity or prior knowledge concerning the subject matter. Adopt an impartial and open-minded approach to listening. Ensure that your responses to them are grounded in factual information.

Please be attentive to the reactions elicited by your responses. In the event that you are posed a question for which you are unprepared to provide an immediate response, it is advisable to express your commitment to sourcing the accurate information and subsequently reaching out to the individual at a later occasion.

6) Refrain from making unwarranted assumptions

One should not presuppose that individuals possess comprehensive knowledge or are familiar with all aspects of the rapidly evolving world. Sexual orientation holds significant weight, and it is imperative that our children receive precise knowledge, communicated with precision and imbued with the principles of self-preservation and respect for others.

By presuming an excess of knowledge on their part, we effectively deprive them of the fundamental understanding necessary for the development of a sound and wholesome concept of sexuality. This implies that it is necessary to begin by comprehending the functioning of our bodies and gaining insight into both the magnificence of affectionate relationships and the capacity for manipulative or exploitative ones.

Do not presuppose that the mere act of questioning denotes their engagement. Many adolescents may pose inquiries regarding sex, sexuality, contraception, and related topics due to their natural curiosity or exposure to information.

Young individuals inquire in order to obtain reliable information or seek clarification. It is imperative that they obtain precise information. Information can serve as an excellent catalyst for initiating engaging discussions.

It should not be presumed that children possess complete comprehension of all information conveyed to them, nor that we possess comprehensive understanding of all their attempts to communicate with us.

It is suggested to consistently encourage adolescents to reiterate and confirm their understanding of the information communicated to them, while also inspiring them to request clarification if needed (and vice versa). If any aspect appears ambiguous, request additional elucidation and be prepared to reiterate and reformulate information in manners that will facilitate their comprehension.

7) Employ various media platforms to generate opportunities for imparting knowledge.

The media nowadays frequently portrays significant amount of sexual content. Television programs, films, online platforms, literary works, and printed publications can serve as effective platforms for imparting knowledge about sexuality to the younger generation.

Moreover, as the narratives predominantly revolve around individuals other than themselves, our adolescent demographic may display a heightened inclination to inquire or provide responses. This is because it entails a discourse regarding individuals unknown to them.

Some of the subjects we should readily be able to locate encompass the origins of offspring, matters concerning romantic allure, considerations regarding LGBTQ matters, customs of courtship, termination of relationships, infatuations, conception, transmission of sexually transmitted diseases, and physiological transformations during adolescence.

Do not deliver a lecture; instead, provide a thorough explanation of the underlying reasons.
Top-down lectures backfire.

It is imperative that we offer our children the necessary support to cultivate the ability to make judicious choices for themselves. By providing instructions or cautioning individuals about severe ramifications through a discourse influenced by emotions, we run the risk of alienating them from ourselves and inadvertently propelling them towards the very behaviors that incite apprehension.

There are two primary factors contributing to the ineffectiveness of lectures. Initially, such explanations possess a tendency towards excessive abstraction whereby they frequently establish intricate associations between a series of actions and a disconcerting consequence.

Furthermore, due to the tendency of adults to deliver lectures amidst intense situations, adolescents are exposed to expressions of anger and perceive feelings of fear, however, they do not derive any advantages from the underlying insights communicated.

We can acquire the skill to present the identical information in a manner that facilitates our adolescents in serenely assimilating the information and permitting it to shape their own conclusions. When youthful individuals independently arrive at conclusions (even with our guidance!), they are more inclined to embrace the solutions and internalize the associated principles.

123

An initial step involves engaging in dialogue rather than making strict requests. It is imperative to communicate to your children that engaging in conversations with them serves as a means of facilitating their development of sound decision-making skills. When imposing expectations upon adolescents, we occasionally prompt them to engage in acts of rebellion.

Conversely, when they possess a lucid comprehension of our objective to ensure their safety and moral upbringing, they express gratitude for both our counsel and the limitations we establish as a framework.

Ensure that your children comprehend the rationale behind your instructions pertaining to sexual conduct. This will facilitate a deeper comprehension among your adolescents regarding your inherent principles and perspectives on sexuality, as well as the rationale behind specific behaviors that contribute to their overall well-being.

Engage in discussions regarding the topic of sex within the broader framework of interpersonal connections, rather than solely presenting it as a means of imparting safety advice. This will also aid them in comprehending the underlying reasons behind your instruction. This course of action will serve to avoid arousing any feelings of control, while simultaneously ensuring that their comprehension of your intentions gravitates towards the notion of safeguarding and nurturing.

9) Depict sexuality as a wholesome and aesthetically pleasing aspect of human existence.

Regrettably, it is all too common that our discussions with our tweens and teens regarding sexual matters revolve primarily around the potential hazards and repercussions of engaging in sexual behavior, neglecting to address the affirmative aspects and emotions associated with such experiences. ty?

Can you recall the sensation of experiencing butterflies in your stomach when you first developed feelings for someone? How about the joy that ensued from the realization that someone whom you held affection for reciprocated those feelings? Alternatively, could one describe the surge of euphoria following an inaugural embrace? It is imperative that we, as responsible adults, communicate to our adolescents regarding the joys and experiences associated with human sexuality.

It is imperative to instill in them a sense of appreciation for their inherent physical attributes, ensuring a comprehensive comprehension of their bodily capabilities and the means to maintain their overall well-being.

One may engage in a conversation with their child regarding the advantages of practicing abstinence, emphasizing not only the physical safety but also the emotional well-being that accompanies this choice. Simultaneously, it is important to address the customary range of emotions that arise during the process of self-discovery and sexual awareness.

Dirty Talk First Steps

Now that you have successfully persuaded yourself that it is permissible to articulate undisclosed longing, we proceed to the initial measures of approaching the matter. While certain individuals find this task effortless, others may still endure a sense of embarrassment due to the potential for rejection or ridicule.

A possible approach to initiate conversation is by sending an insinuating message to your partner, allowing you to gauge their reaction.

You can also followup with a "dirty phone call" even if your lover is nearby — if he or she is interested in you may find yourself coupled soon!

Let us explore alternative categories of alluring textual exchanges or telephonic communication. Certainly, you have the option to modify any of these options or create countless alternatives. This marks the initiation of a novel and alluring form of communication.

SEXY MEMORIES

Each individual possesses an initial recollection or perception of the occasion when they were first acquainted or encountered their romantic partner. Presented below are a selection of conversational prompts that could initiate a stimulating dialogue.

I recall the moment when I initially laid eyes upon you by the pool—I harbored a strong attraction towards you at that instant!

Upon initially encountering you at the establishment, I observed, "Your smile is pleasant and your physique is appealing."

Upon our initial encounter, I found myself inquisitive about the contents concealed within your denim trousers...

◆ ◆ ◆

Engaging in flirtatious behavior with a hint of naughtiness.

As an example, suppose you have completed your occupational tasks for the day and now find yourself in the confines of your residence without any company. "You are aware that your partner will be returning home imminently." Presented below are a selection of playfully suggestive messages that can be sent to elicit a heightened sense of excitement in the recipient. With the utilization of these, one can engage in playful banter and subsequently satisfy to one's heart's content.

I appreciate the aesthetic appeal of how your posterior appears in the jeans that I have procured for you.

Your fragrance entices me to nestle my visage in the strands of your hair.

I have an unexpected revelation prepared for you this evening.

The fragrance you're wearing is so captivating, it entices me to lean closer and appreciate its alluring aroma.

The level of excitement I feel in anticipation of your return to our residence is so immense that it might result in my attire becoming inadequate.

I possess a blindfold, a feather, and a container of lubricant — return to our place and let us engage in imaginative explorations.

If you demonstrate proper behavior, I will grant you the opportunity to engage in more mischievous activities at a later time.

I have engaged in outdoor activities and now I require a warm bath. Could you kindly assist me with reaching those challenging areas, please?

Upon your arrival at your residence, we could partake in an engaging pursuit in search of hidden treasures. I have placed a map on the kitchen table to provide guidance toward the concealed treasure. I would like to offer a subtle suggestion that the treasure can be found in the bedroom.

◆◆◆

NON-JUDGMENTAL ENVIRONMENT (WHERE YOU CAN EXPRESS YOUR COMPLAINTS IN PRIVATE) LIMITLESS SPACE OF ACCEPTANCE (WHERE YOU ARE FREE TO VENT AND EXPRESS YOUR FRUSTRATIONS IN PRIVATE)

In an environment of trust, one's intimate relations should be exempt from any form of criticism or evaluation. During intense moments, one cannot predict the utterances that may emerge from one's own or their partner's lips.

In the majority of instances, if one maintains trust in oneself and in their partner, circumstances tend to turn out favorably. In the event that an individual within this group utters a discomforting remark, it is advisable to dismiss it with minimal concern and proceed to engage in more enjoyable discourse.

The act of delving into language and communication will yield substantial benefits, not only in the present moment but also in your long-term recollection of the intimacy and passion you experienced.

❖❖❖

Certain individuals prefer warm temperatures, while others have a preference for even higher levels of heat.

The container of affection shall be infused with passionate and suggestive messages you have dispatched — allow me to present a few additional ones to intensify the ardor!

Do you prefer the lights to be turned off or on when I express my desire for intimacy with you?

The position known as "doggy style" provides an immensely pleasurable experience when engaged with you.

I derive immense joy from observing your countenance upon your arrival.

Observing your arrival is an exceptionally stimulating experience.

I derive immense pleasure from experiencing your presence within me.

I experience heightened arousal when I observe you engaging in oral stimulation with me.

I plan to engage in intimate activities with you throughout the entire night, stimulating your senses until you experience climax.

◆◆◆

THAT HITS THE SPOT

We collectively appreciate receiving affirmative feedback and value constructive criticism as well. Naturally, one would employ their own language in the midst of intense emotions, nevertheless, presented below are a few recommendations on effectively directing your partner and expressing gratitude for their admirable efforts.

Right there!

Indeed, that is commendable.

Don't you dare stop!

You can exert even greater effort.

Deeper!

I'm nearly there!

I am fond of that.

Harder!

Don't stop!

Right there!

Keep doing that!

Oh right there!

If this pace persists, I will imminently reach climax.

Does that feel good?

This sensation is quite pleasing, wouldn't you agree?

Just like that baby!

Please continue, as this sensation is truly remarkable — may you sense the intense moisture within me?

Are you able to perceive the extent of the burden I am experiencing due to your actions?

You arouse me greatly.

Chapter 7: Practicing Responsible Digital Communication in the Context of Relationships

Similar to any other action or manifestation, there exist guidelines of appropriate etiquette. There exist certain guidelines that should be adhered to when engaging in the practice of sexting. In the following chapter, you will familiarize yourself with the appropriate and inappropriate practices related to the act of sexting.

In the contemporary era that we inhabit, it is a rarity to encounter an individual devoid of a mobile phone, and even less likely to come across someone unfamiliar with the art of text messaging. Elevate this situation further and subsequently inquire about the quantity of individuals aged 18 to 50 who have abstained from sending their partner a risqué text message. The majority of individuals are aware of this particular mode of prelude.

Notwithstanding any amusement derived from it, it is crucial to bear in mind that engaging in sexting can be perilous if not conducted in the appropriate manner or with a suitable person. Engaging in sexting with someone outside of your committed relationship has the potential to cause harm and may even lead to the deterioration of various aspects of your life. In response to a highly debated question, it is indeed considered a form of infidelity to engage in sexting with an individual when you are already in a committed relationship. It is a prelude to sexual activity.

The Dos

Start Slowly

There is no need to hasten foreplay; hence, it is advisable to refrain from rushing into sexting. It embodies a distinctive variant of this category of entertainment, and it is widely recognized that hastily engaging in prelude activities is unfavorable. It represents a gradual accumulation of anticipation. Engage in playful banter and friendly teasing, reserving the more substantial aspects of the conversation for later on. You will not find cause for remorse by pursuing this course of action.

Engage in activities with an individual whom you have confidence in.

Engaging in sexually explicit conversations with individuals you have not witnessed in an unclothed state or had limited communication with is not a prudent course of action. Sexting should be limited to individuals with whom you have established trust and a genuine connection. Failing to do so would leave you with no one but yourself to hold accountable should your explicit images be circulated to acquaintances via email.

Engage in intimate communication when you are physically separated.

Whether you are temporarily absent due to a prior commitment or you are traveling for professional purposes, engaging in intimate communication through digital means presents a remarkable opportunity to maintain the passionate connection during your absence. Kindly inform your significant other that you constantly have them in your thoughts, and the anticipation of your reunion is beyond your imagination.

Remember to Press Delete

While reminiscing about the messages can provide enjoyment, the gratification quickly dissipates when an intrusive individual seizes control of your mobile device. Please ensure the conversation is purged upon its completion. Delete, delete, delete!

Use Auto Correct

A communication that contains numerous misspellings is highly disengaging. You appear to lack intelligence, and it is highly probable that the other individual will dismiss your opinion without much consideration. If you are uncertain about the spelling of a word, it is advisable to refrain from utilizing it. Substitute or employ your auto correct feature to enhance your intelligence.

The Don'ts

Sexting Someone Unknown

Refrain from engaging in explicit messaging with individuals whom you have not personally witnessed in a state of undress. It has the potential to create a highly uncomfortable and frequently unwelcome predicament. Engage in verbal banter and reserve the visual aspects for a later stage of the relationship. The young lady is not interested in viewing a depiction of your male reproductive organ, gentlemen. Convey to her romantic sentiments through written expressions.

Engage in verbal communication that you would refrain from uttering directly to the individuals involved.

One advantage of engaging in sexting is the inability to visually perceive the individual's countenance. There are no reactions that one should feel ashamed or humiliated about. Nevertheless, it can backfire when your partner requests you to utter it in the midst of the act. This implies that if you are capable of sending a message via text, you must also possess the ability to articulate the same words face-to-face.

Use a Work Phone

It is imperative that personal communication be conveyed exclusively through one's personal mobile device. Unforeseen circumstances may arise, resulting in potential repercussions on one's employment status. This is a matter of common knowledge; nevertheless, it has occurred on multiple occasions.

Please submit the photographs featuring your face.

It is strongly advised to refrain from transmitting images that reveal your facial features or any distinctive characteristics of your physique. In the eventuality of the image being observed, one's identity shall remain anonymous.

Forget the Age Limits

It is imperative to always remember that sexting is an activity intended for individuals who are at least 18 years of age or older. Engaging in sexting by either party is deemed inappropriate and should cease without delay.

Retrieve numerical data from social media sources.

It is strongly advised against seeking out the contact information of an individual discovered on a social media platform and engaging in explicit communication with them. It is imperative that you engage in a preliminary discussion beforehand. This individual needs to familiarize themselves with you, and it must be acknowledged that it would be somewhat intrusive if you were to actively search for their contact information without their explicit consent. If such an occurrence transpires, one may resort to pursuing legal remedies.

Ask for Pictures

If you lack personal acquaintance or are not involved in an intimate connection, abstain from requesting pictures specifically showcasing the chest region. Numerous women receive such requests, arousing feelings of anger within them. You shall never obtain the photographs, therefore refrain from attempting to do so.

Type Orgasms

Sending explicit text messages is impolite and uncomfortable. Please refrain from transmitting expressions such as "ooooh" or "aaauuggh." It is perceived as demonstrating a lack of intelligence. Moreover, how can one experience orgasmic pleasure whilst engaging in the act of typing?

The Significance Of Enjoyment

If laughter has never been shared amidst the intimate moments, it is opportune to adopt a more lighthearted approach. It is essential to acquire the ability to let go of inhibitions in each other's presence. While you may be questioning the relation between this topic and explicit communication, it is undeniably relevant. If one approaches lovemaking with such unwavering seriousness, to the point where mutual relaxation and the pursuit of pleasure are neglected, the vast potential and benefits that intimate encounters hold may be greatly compromised.

Engaging in the enjoyable endeavor of jointly perusing the esteemed literary work, Kama Sutra, and faithfully experimenting with its varied techniques has the potential to significantly alter the trajectory of your intimate relations. Participating in this activity promises amusement, and the joviality you express will pave the way for subsequent experiences. Addressing you, who possesses prominent breasts, can serve as an element that you both partake in during your enjoyable moments. It's intimate. Others do not refer to you by that name, and you are aware that when he utilizes this appellation, it signifies his seriousness towards the matter. Engage in the exploration of affection and humor, for in doing so, you can alleviate tension and enhance the quality of your intimate experiences. The entire purpose behind employing language to articulate one's emotions or desires lies in its ability to enhance sexual stimulation and generate a truly exhilarating experience.

A gentleman who artfully expresses his desire for his partner's pleasure and invites her to surrender to his passionate advances can be deemed highly alluring and enjoyable to spend time with. Furthermore, she can anticipate with eagerness his plans to accomplish precisely that. Consider the scenario in which a woman confidently positions herself above her spouse while he attends to household tasks, openly revealing her intimate regions and expressing her readiness and anticipation, thus enticing him in that very moment. Have you considered abstaining from wearing undergarments while attending a restaurant and granting him an exclusive and discreet prelude? It is undeniably enticing and your audacious demeanor may sufficiently pique his interest in returning home. If fortunate, he might secure accommodations at a hotel or offer transportation in a vehicle. What occurs within the confines of your relationship is a matter strictly relegated to the two individuals involved.

The enjoyment experienced during intimate moments need not cease merely due to the presence of children. A significant number of women opt for nightwear as they prefer to maintain their modesty in the presence of their children. You cannot indefinitely rely on this as an excuse, nor should you. Exposing one's nakedness holds a certain significance; however, for individuals who have offspring, perhaps considering engaging in an intimate escapade with one's partner during the hours when the children are attending school, and employing unconventional methods to stimulate him through unexpected provocation:

If you return to our residence promptly, I am eagerly anticipating your arrival in an unclad state.

Hello, my darling. Would you be interested in engaging in intimate relations?

Merely being married and assuming adult responsibilities does not signify the demise of the inner-child. Elder individuals continue to engage in explicit language and should be afforded the right to do so. Have fun with it. Display courage and confidence in your interactions with your partner, ensuring that they understand that your boldness is exclusively directed towards them. In doing so, no negative consequences shall arise.

Enter the room while he is ablution. Please disrobe and enter the shower. Are you interested in assisting me with lathering soap on my body? This may elicit certain thoughts in his mind, particularly given his state of undress, where his immediate reaction becomes apparent. The key lies in cultivating a state of utmost comfort with your partner, wherein no restrictions or limitations apply - quite literally.

The enjoyment experienced within the confines of the bedroom can extend beyond those boundaries. Dress in his preferred low cut sweater and present his lunch in a enticing manner while maintaining a composed demeanor. Engage in playful banter, cater to his desires, and explore amusing colloquialisms together that alleviate the potential offense associated with their usage, as both of you acknowledge the lighthearted nature of the interaction and have no intention of causing harm to anyone.

CHAPTER FIVE: AVAN

I had grown tired of this nonsensical situation.

My heart palpitated vigorously within my thoracic cavity, while my abdominal region embraced a taut configuration. Did I perceive him affirm that I was his partner?

What was his intended meaning behind that statement?

Recognizing the presence of an inexplicable phenomenon, I proceeded to descend the tree.

Perhaps it was not prudent, but I intended to approach him directly for a confrontation.

I was experiencing heightened nervous sensations emanating in various directions, yet I desired to obtain answers.

Although he was largely unfamiliar to me, my intuition reassured me that he had no intention of causing harm. Nicholas provided assistance to me on a previous occasion, during my hiking expedition.

Moreover, he had explicitly stated that he was apprehending me on fraudulent grounds, which was highly unfortunate.

However, I was irresistibly attracted to him.

Had a taxi appeared at that precise moment and extended an offer for transportation, I would have declined the opportunity to distance myself from his presence.

Stupid? Maybe.

However, my intention was to remain with him until I had obtained clarity regarding the situation.

Upon commencing my descent from the tree, Nicholas proceeded to elevate his arms. "Be careful," he said.

He was the individual responsible for causing me to climb the tree, and now he desired to assume the role of an overly protective hero?

No thanks.

I shouted, commanding you to distance yourself from the tree.

With a hint of hesitance, he receded slightly, yet he remained in close proximity.

Upon reaching the ground, I promptly brushed off my hands and gestured towards him. I kindly request that you provide me with an explanation of the current circumstances. I appropriated a substantial branch and positioned it before my person. "Right now."

I would like to extend my sincerest apologies for my behavior. Typically, I take pride in my ability to effectively embody the responsibilities of the sheriff of this town. Regrettably, today proved to be an exception to this notion."

I perceived a sudden elevation of my eyebrows. Okay. That was a start. "Yes. Your conduct was deplorable.

He nodded. If you would be amenable to accompanying me to the residence, we could engage in a dialogue.

I require further clarification before proceeding with you.

Nicholas extended his hand. There exist serpents within this vicinity. And remnants of a previous barbed-wire barrier. Would it be possible for us to stroll back to the road, at the very least?

"Okay. But you go first. I'll follow."

He appeared displeased with the situation, yet he proceeded to walk ahead of me. I could perceive that he remained cognizant of my every action.

"I was overcome with a brief lapse in judgement," Nicholas stated.

"You did," I said. I unintentionally placed my foot upon a twig, and experienced a heightened state of alarm as it emitted a resounding crack.

I halted momentarily and retrieved the stick, passing my hand along the rough surface of the bark. I have never had particularly superior auditory capabilities. Throughout the law school lectures, I was required to occupy a seat in close proximity to the front in the classrooms designed in an auditorium-style format. My auditory acuity appeared to be at a modest level, if not subpar.

At present, the audible sound of a bee's buzzing reached my ears.

Nicholas appeared to be regarding me with a curious expression.

"Avan? "Are you feeling alright?" Nicholas inquired.

"I am in satisfactory condition." I released the stick and commenced walking. The intense gaze directed towards me by him was unnerving, albeit somewhat intriguing.

We ultimately resumed our progress and in due course arrived at the roadway. I was experiencing the sensation of thirst and fatigue, accompanied by discomfort in my stomach. I cast my gaze upon my abdominal region. Although there was no evidence of blood, my utmost desire was to recline and rest.

Nausea washed over me.

"I believe it would be preferable for me to return to your residence after all," I expressed. Dammit. Now I was dizzy. I extended my hands, sensing an imminent forward inclination that would result in a face-first descent should I proceed further. I inhaled deeply, drawing in the invigorating air, in the hopes of restoring my equilibrium.

It appeared that he immediately took notice. He advanced, positioning himself in proximity without making physical contact.

I was unwilling to assume the role of a helpless individual under his protection, darn it. Although I may possess a lesser stature in comparison to his, I have always been self-sufficient and have never relied upon a man for my rescue, nor do I have any intentions of doing so at present.

However, there was an undeniable allure in his act of rescuing me. He appeared remarkably attractive as he stood amidst the expanse of the field, bathed in the soft glow of the declining sun. He displayed apprehension regarding my well-being.

How could I harbor any resentment towards that?

"You sustained injuries a mere few hours prior," Nicholas stated. "You need to rest. Furthermore, sustenance and hydration are required."

I agreed. The only sustenance I had consumed were a small portion of peanut butter that I had obtained from the residence of that eccentric individual.

"Okay. "I have currently recovered." On this occasion, I permitted him to accompany me, staying in close proximity. It would have elicited amusement had it not possessed such an extraordinarily peculiar nature. Despite its strangeness, there was an undeniable allure to it.

Nicholas extended his arm and gently placed his hand on the lower region of my back.

I also did not coerce him into relocating it.

We proceeded at a leisurely pace due to my deliberate tempo, and ultimately, we arrived at the residence.

I had failed to give it appropriate notice previously, but it possessed an admirable ambiance. The structure was constructed with white siding and embellished with stone accents, featuring a spacious wooden porch. In the vicinity, a number of dwellings akin to it could be observed.

The setting bore a striking resemblance to a suburban enclave within a sprawling neighborhood, rather than an isolated rural area in the distant countryside.

Nicholas opened the door.

A refreshing breeze enveloped me, prompting my entrance.

Nicholas smoothly pulled a chair away from the table and took his seat. I will fetch you a glass of water.

Subsequent to his act of pouring, I received the glass with deep gratitude.

Subsequently, Nicholas presented me with a plate containing a portioned apple accompanied by cheese and crackers. I consumed them expeditiously, subsequently attaining a state of preparedness. I was compelled to exercise patience no further.

"Okay. I kindly request an explanation of the current situation."

He took his seat beside me at the table, yet remained silent. Well, that was ominous. It appeared that I would be compelled to assume responsibility and handle the situation on my own.

Nicholas, I encountered you during a hiking expedition. I am cognizant of having witnessed your transformation into a lupine creature, or a similar entity. Subsequently, you pursued me and assumed the role of apprehending me, although in reality, you abducted me. So I think you owe me an explanation."

Instructing Adolescent Males On Sexual Education And Interpersonal Connections.

Young adults, particularly adolescent males, often perceive sexual conquest as a means of attaining social status. They have acquired knowledge about it through the media and received information through their acquaintances. You are required to elucidate to him the fallacy of this claim and reassure him that it is possible to maintain both a composed demeanor and a state of virginity as a father. Kindly convey to him that it is commonplace for numerous adolescents to experience a lack of readiness for sexual activities. It is imperative to ensure that your child comprehends the concept of "readiness" as numerous adolescents nowadays partake in sexual behavior prior to being prepared.

Adolescents acquire knowledge about sexism and the objectification of women through exposure to the media, representing a disheartening facet of contemporary society. Please reflect upon the desired behavior for your son in his interactions with his partners. Please notify him that it is imperative to treat girls and women, including any prospective partners, with utmost respect, refraining from regarding them as mere objects of vanity or status. Engaging in coercive sexual advances and objectifying a woman for one's own gratification both display a lack of respect. Instruct him to refrain from pursuing further if his spouse manifests any indication of doubt or hesitation pertaining to any aspect of their physical engagement.

Presently, it is imperative to ensure that your son possesses a thorough understanding of the definition of rape. Ensure that you effectively communicate to him that the word "no" is universally definitive, emphasizing the importance of refraining from exploiting or disregarding a woman who may be incapable of voicing her objection. Respect is the foremost consideration.

It is important for you to recognize that it is highly probable that your son will partake in sexual activity prior to your perceived readiness or preferred timeframe. You must ensure his preparedness as a consequence. Consistently emphasize the importance of condom usage to him and maintain a resolute stance in expressing your viewpoint. Notify him about the various contraceptive alternatives and their corresponding rates of effectiveness.

Finally, it is imperative to actively maintain honesty when discussing matters relating to sexually transmitted diseases and infections with him. This encompasses providing accurate information regarding their modes of transmission, visual manifestations, and appropriate timings for medical screening. The mature and accountable approach towards engaging in sexual activity is to prioritize one's personal safety. If an individual is not prepared to prioritize safety, it indicates that they are not prepared for engaging in sexual activity.

Engaging in sexual activity should be limited to individuals who are involved in a sincere and long-term partnership based on love and commitment. It is imperative that your adolescent son be promptly informed of this matter, however, the discussion must persist. It is imperative that he comprehends the importance of requiring respectful behavior towards his partners and recognizes that engaging in sexual activity should not be regarded as a symbol of social standing. If he has not engaged in sexual activity as of now or if he chooses to abstain, he should not be labeled as a failure. However, if he does not wish to defer until he reaches adulthood, he must grasp the concept of maintaining personal safety and comprehend the importance of taking necessary precautions. This is a highly consequential dialogue that holds considerable significance, as it represents one of the most pivotal discussions you will engage in with your adolescent son. Therefore, it is imperative that you approach this exchange with utmost sincerity and candor.

A significant challenge faced by numerous individuals when it comes to parenting is the task of raising adolescents. The preservation of discipline becomes increasingly challenging, occasionally appearing unattainable. Determining the appropriate timing for imposing limitations and permitting liberties, being flexible yet resolute, intervening while also allowing space, presents a considerable challenge.

A challenging aspect to navigate often pertains to the realm of communication. It can prove to be a challenge to possess the knowledge of what to express, the appropriate timing for its delivery, and the suitable manner in which to articulate it. As your adolescent reaches the stage of initiating romantic relationships, the complexity of these conversations and choices becomes increasingly intricate.

As the conclusion of Teen Dating Violence Awareness Month approaches, we wish to emphasize the utmost importance of parental involvement in both mitigating instances of teen dating violence and cultivating relationships that are characterized by sound emotional well-being.

If you happen to be a parent to an adolescent in the process of maturing, it would be prudent to consider imparting these significant subjects pertaining to relationships to your male offspring prior to his foray into the realm of romantic engagements:

Kindly elucidate the defining characteristics of a prosperous interpersonal bond.

Please ensure that you provide your adolescent with comprehensive guidance regarding the essential principles of a healthy and stable interpersonal connection. Outline how respect, mutual comprehension, trustworthiness, integrity, effective communication, and assistance serve as the fundamental pillars of a robust and flourishing interpersonal bond.

It is imperative that both parties in a relationship establish and diligently maintain appropriate boundaries that promote health and balance. A reliable companion will embrace your authentic self, demonstrate regard for your choices, and recognize your achievements. Moreover, a robust partnership refrains from imposing limitations on the personal liberties of either individual, granting both partners the autonomy to pursue their own outside interests and maintain friendships.